D1117204

DIRTY JAYNE

Amy Mitchell

Illustrated by Jean Spencer

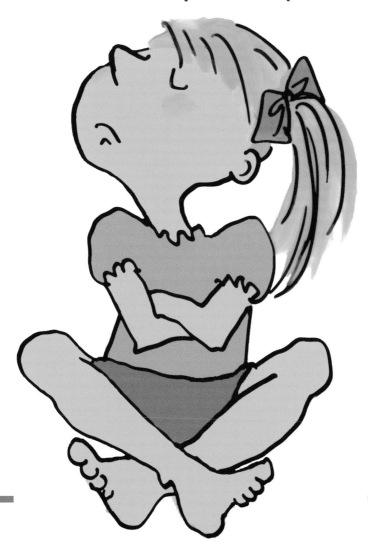

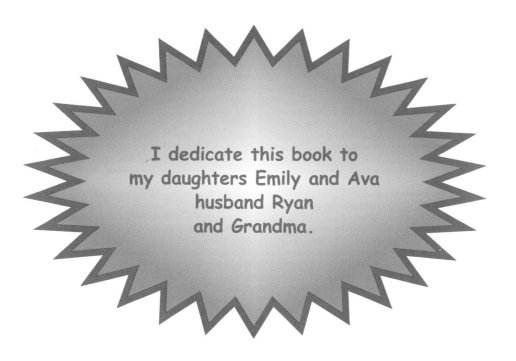

I dedicate this book to
my daughters Emily and Ava
husband Ryan
and Grandma.

Mayhaven Publishing, Inc.
P O Box 557
Mahomet, IL 61853
USA

All rights reserved.
No part of this book may be reproduced or transmitted in any form
or by any means without written permission from the author,
except for the inclusion of brief quotations in a review.

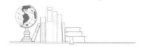

Illustrations by Jean Spencer
Copyright © 2011 Amy Mitchell
Library of Congress Cataloging Number: 2011938403
First Edition—First Printing 2011
ISBN 13 978 1932278798
ISBN 10 1932278796

Dirty Jayne was a little girl
who never liked to bathe.

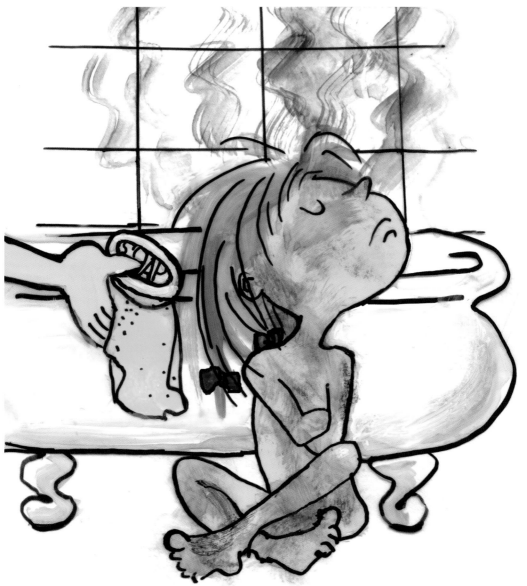

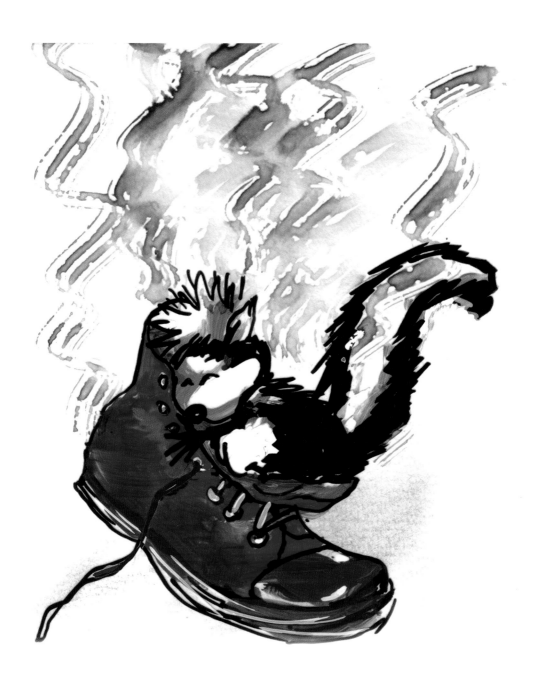

"If you don't bathe, you'll stink worse
than a skunk in sweaty gym shoes,"
her mother warned her after
days of Jayne not bathing.

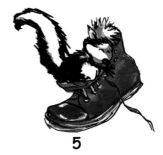

"Yes," agreed her father.
"If you don't bathe,
you'll stink worse than rotten eggs
in a pot of sour cream,
and no one will ever want to
play with you."

But Jayne would still not take a bath.

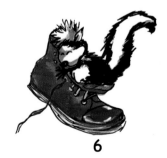

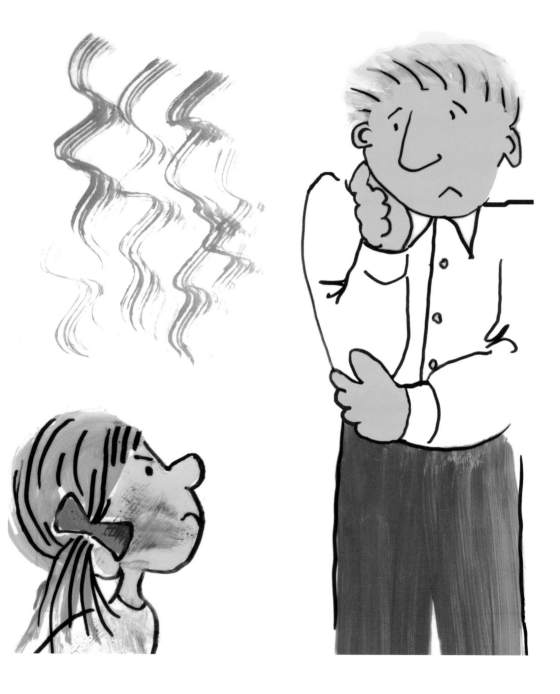

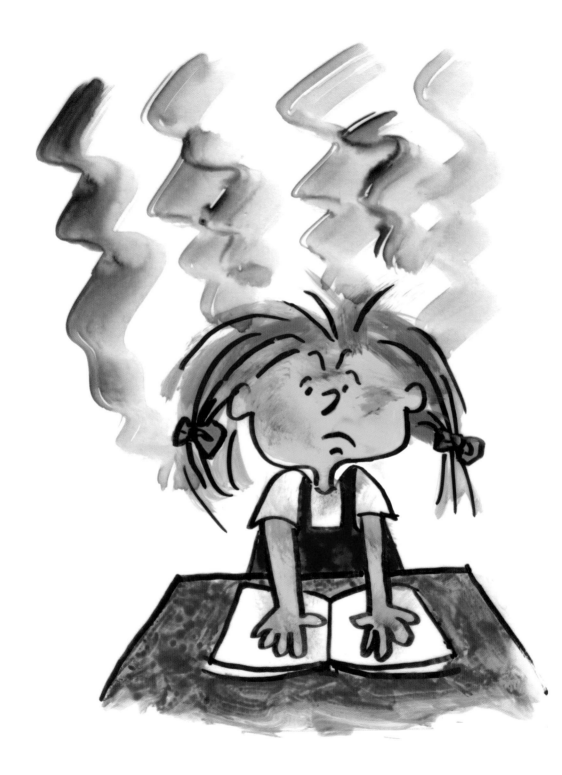

Days went by.
Jayne didn't wash.
She stopped brushing her teeth.
She stopped combing her hair.
She stopped trimming her nails.

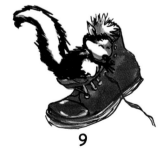

Just as her parents warned,
Jayne began to smell so awful,
none of the students in her class
would play with her at recess.

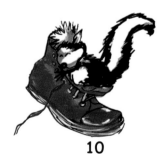

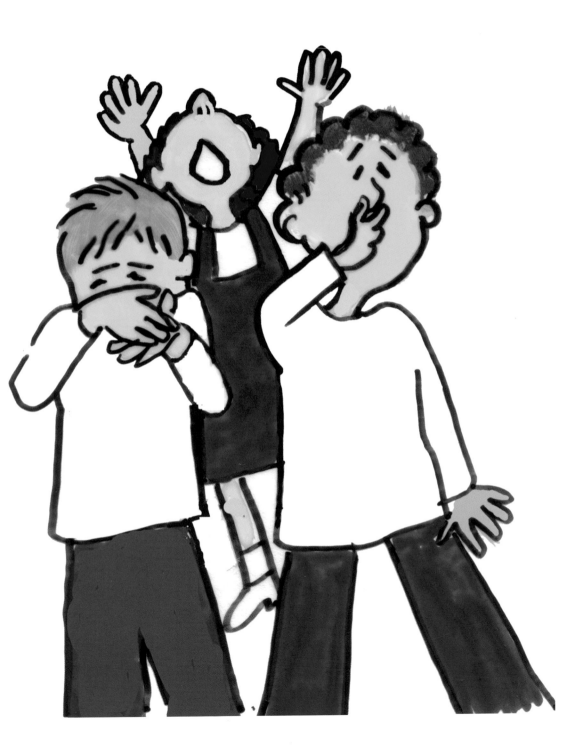

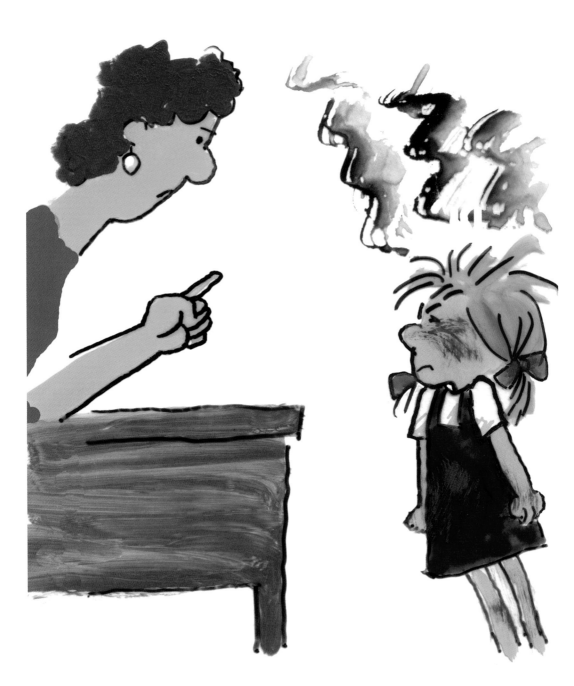

Then, one day, the teacher called
Jayne to her desk.
"Jayne," she said, "I'm afraid that
if you don't shower
you won't be allowed back to our class.
Quite frankly, your stinky smell
is distracting everyone from learning."

But Jayne would not take a shower.

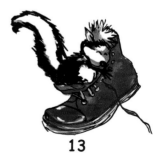

Weeks passed.
Jayne's smiling face became
covered in dirt,
and when she grinned,
bugs waved hello from inside her mouth.

But Jayne would still not take a bath.

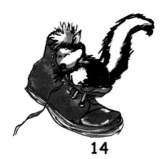

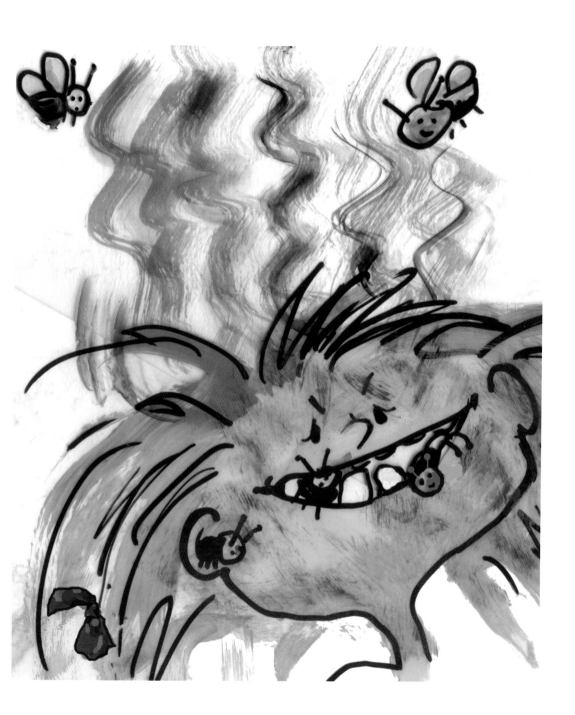

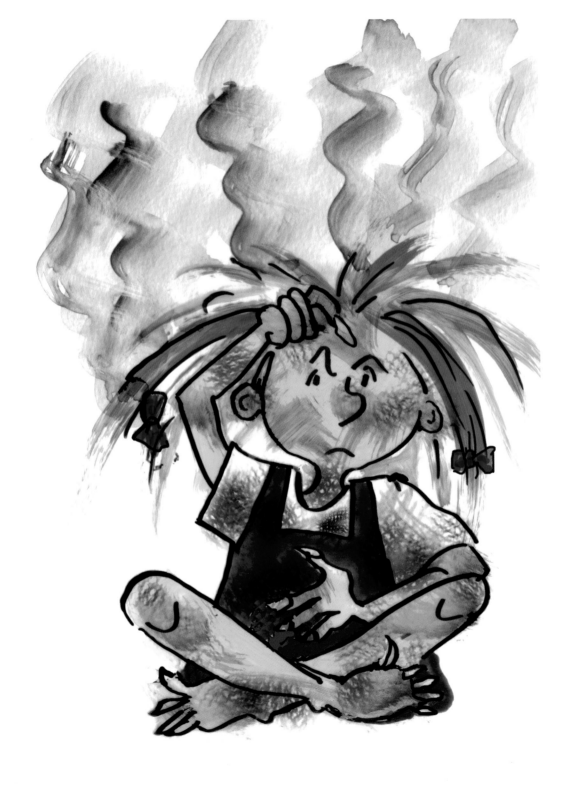

She never even changed her clothes.
Her fingernails grew so long,
they began to curl at the tips.

Soon, Jayne's body began
to itch all over.

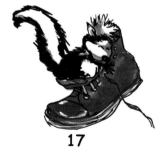

Frustrated, her mother dragged
her to the tub of warm bubbly water,
but Jayne would not
even wash a single toe!

Her father took away
Jayne's toys, one by one,

but Jayne would still not take a bath.

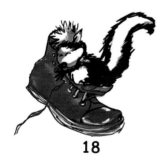

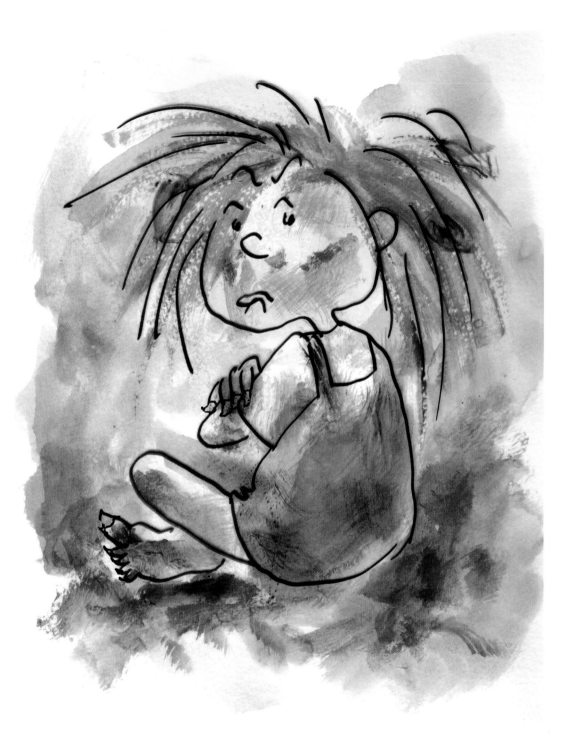

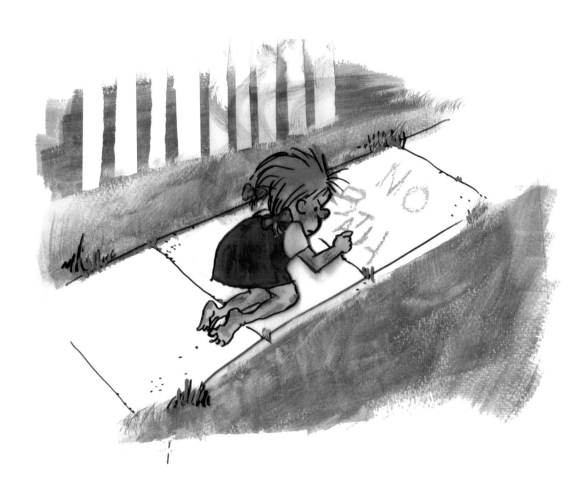

Months went by.
Soon, the whole town could smell
the stink of Dirty Jayne.
Even though her parents
were embarrassed,

Jayne would still not take
a bath or shower.

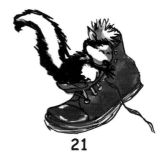

Then, one day,
when the stink of Jayne
became unbearable,
her mother and father banished her
to the backyard
with a bar of soap and a water hose,
locking the door behind her.

"You can't come back inside," they said,
"until you take a shower!"

But Jayne would still not get clean.

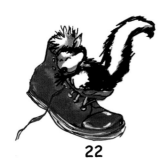

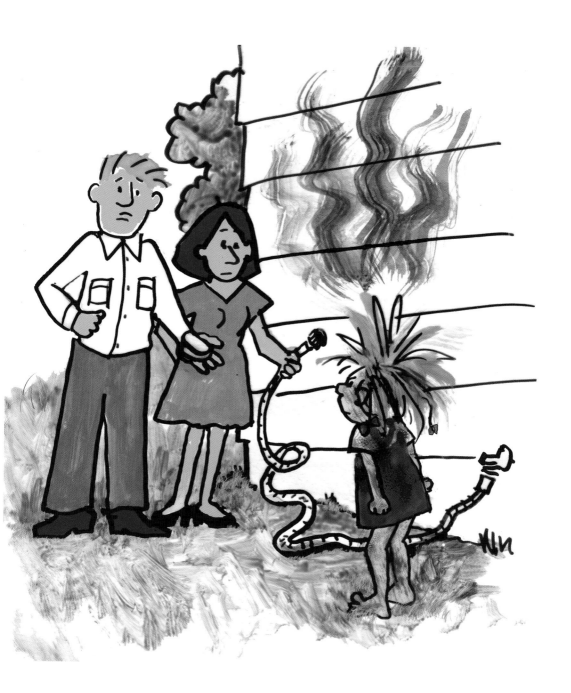

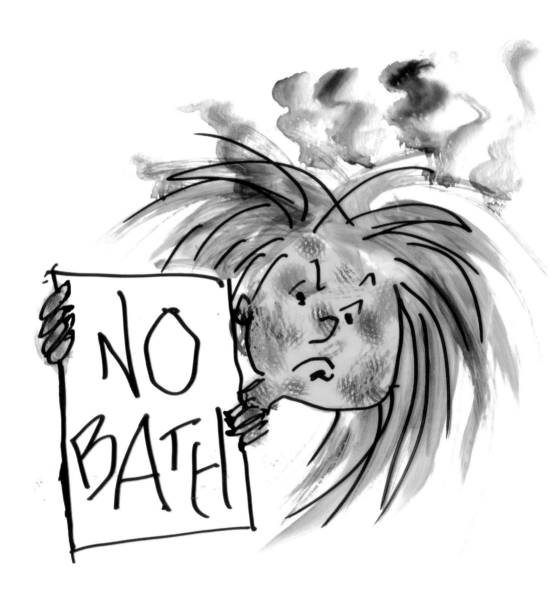

Instead, Jayne sat in that
backyard for days
enjoying the smell of her filth.
She rolled in mud.
She jumped in the leaves.
She slept in a pile of dust.

She just got dirtier,
and dirtier and dirtier.

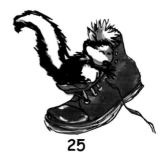

One day, it suddenly grew too cold
to be outside.
The soap began to freeze.
The water in the hose slowly
turned to ice.

Now, Jayne could not take a bath.

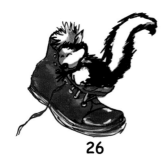

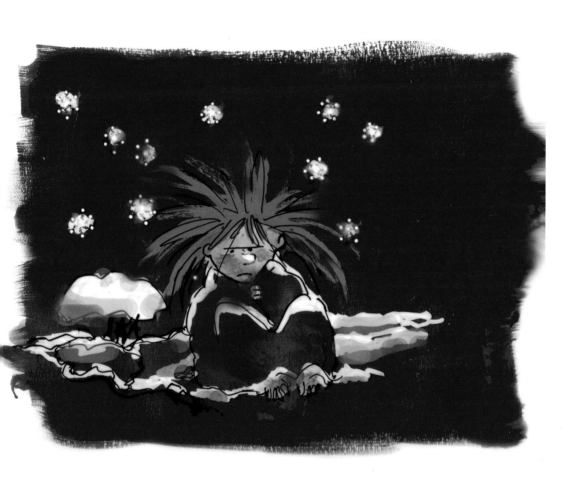

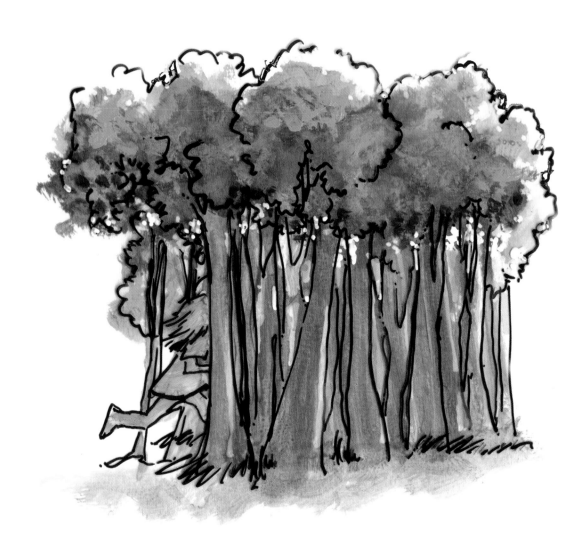

So one day she ran into the woods
and disappeared,
leaving nothing
but a linger of stink behind her.

Jayne was never ever seen again.

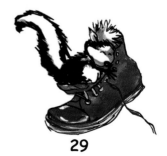

Some say Jayne is still in that woods,
waiting for another
stinky friend to join her.
Some say she met a boy
named Dirty Jym
who spirited her away.

But I say, you better keep clean,
because if you don't
then Jayne might smell you,
and if she does, well then, good luck.

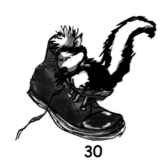

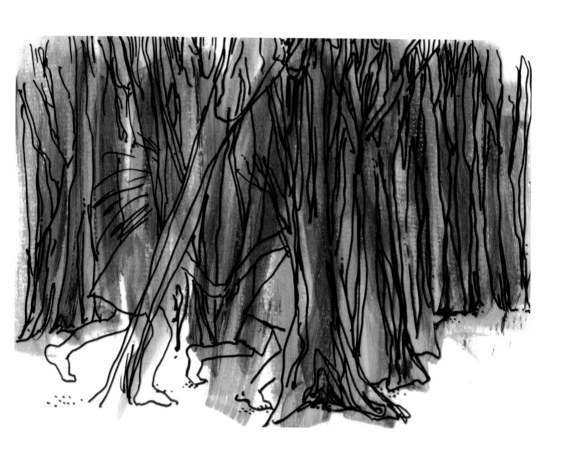

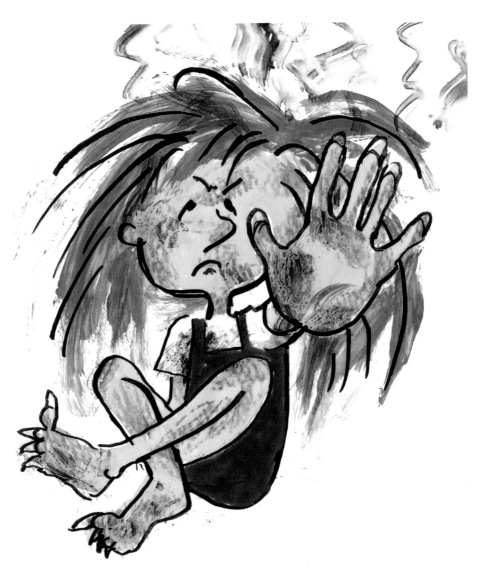

At least you know I warned you...